Why You're Tired, Fat, and Foggy

(And What to Do About It)

Steven E. Warren, MD, DPA

and Darren Lopez, MBA

Regenerative Wellness Center

Salt Lake City area, Utah

Why You're Tired, Fat, and Foggy (And What to Do About It)

ISBN: 978-1-972800-01-0

Published by Regenerative Wellness Center

Salt Lake City area, Utah

Second printing, 2026.

Medical disclaimer: This book is for general education. It is not a substitute for medical care, diagnosis, or treatment. Talk to your own physician before making changes to medication, supplementation, or lifestyle.

A Note Before We Start

After forty-five years of seeing patients, the most common thing I hear is this: I am tired all the time and nobody can tell me why. I wrote this book for those patients.

This book is the simple version. There is a bigger book called The Living Chip that goes deep into the science. It is written for doctors and serious science readers. This is not that book. This book is for everyone else. The person who is tired and does not know why. The person whose doctor says you are fine but who does not feel fine.

Everything in here is based on real science. I just took out the parts that make your eyes glaze over and replaced them with cartoons.

Dr. Steve

Foundation First

What Is Foundation First?

Foundation First is the protocol I built in my practice after forty-five yea
of seeing the same pattern. Patients sent to specialist after specialist. Prescribed expensive therapy after expensive therapy. While the foundations stay broken. Sleep is wrecked. Nutrition is wrecked. Movement is gone. Stress is unmanaged. Labs say everything is fine.

Foundation First fixes the base before anything else. Sleep, food, movement, alcohol and stress, basic labs, hormones, mitochondrial health. In that order. No peptides, no IVs, no fancy interventions until th
foundation is solid.

Most patients do not need the fancy stuff. Most patients need the foundation.

This book is the patient-facing entry point into the Foundation First protocol. The 90-Day Reboot in Chapter 10 is the protocol in action.

How to Read This Book

- Read it in order. Each chapter builds on the one before.
- Look at the cartoons. They teach the concepts.
- Read The Simple Version box at the end of each chapter.
- Do the 90-Day Reboot in Chapter 10.

Contents

Chapter 1

You're a Computer (No, Seriously)

Most patients sitting across from me feel tired, foggy, and slow, and the truth is the cells inside of them are running on low battery.

That's not a joke. Every single cell in your body works like a little computer. It takes in information. It processes it. It sends out signals. It builds things, breaks things down, and repairs itself. Just like a computer, it needs power to do all of this.

The power comes from tiny machines inside your cells called mitochondria. Say it like this: my-toe-CON-dree-uh. Think of them as the power plants of your body.

You have thousands of these power plants in every single cell. Your heart cells have about 5,000 each, because your heart never stops working. Your brain cells have about 2,000 each, because thinking takes a lot of energy. Even your fat cells have mitochondria, they need power to burn fat.

Here's the problem.

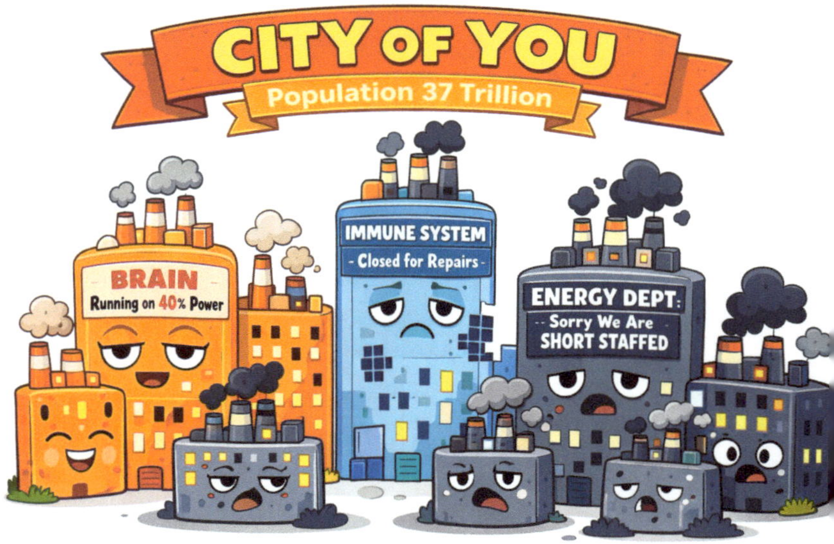
CITY OF YOU
Population 37 Trillion
BRAIN
Running on 40% Power
IMMUNE SYSTEM
- Closed for Repairs -
ENERGY DEPT:
-- Sorry We Are
SHORT STAFFED

These power plants get old. They get rusty. They slow down. And when they slow down, everything in your body slows down with them.

Your brain gets foggy. Your energy crashes after lunch. Your belly stores more fat. Your immune system gets lazy. Your mood drops. Your joints ache. Your sleep gets worse.

Most people go to the doctor and say, "I'm tired all the time." The doctor runs some tests. Everything comes back "normal." The doctor says, "You're fine."

But you're not fine. You're running at 60% power and nobody checked the power plants.

The City of You

Think of it this way. Imagine your body is a city. A big, busy city with millions of buildings. Each building is a cell. Inside each building is a generator that keeps the lights on, the heat running, and the computers working.

Now imagine that half of those generators are old, leaky, and running out of fuel. The lights start to flicker. The heat goes in and out. The computers crash in the middle of the day.

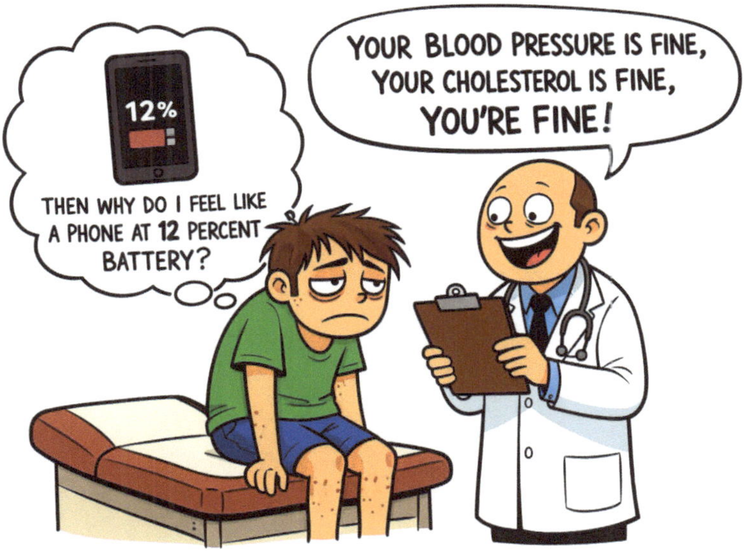
12%
THEN WHY DO I FEEL LIKE A PHONE AT 12 PERCENT BATTERY?
YOUR BLOOD PRESSURE IS FINE, YOUR CHOLESTEROL IS FINE, YOU'RE FINE!

What happens? People in the city start complaining. "It's cold." "The internet is slow." "Nothing works." Somebody calls the mayor and says, "This city is falling apart."

But nobody checks the generators.

That's what's happening in your body right now. Your cells are the buildings. Your mitochondria are the generators. And nobody, not your doctor, not your trainer, not the label on your multivitamin, is checking to see if the generators are actually working.

What Your Power Plants Make Every time your mitochondria do their job, they make something called ATP. Think of ATP as energy money. Everything your body does costs ATP.

• Beating your heart: costs ATP. • Blinking your eyes: costs ATP. • Thinking a thought: costs ATP. • Digesting your lunch: costs ATP. • Fighting off a cold: costs ATP. • Burning belly fat: costs ATP. You spend about 88 pounds of ATP every single day. That's not a typo, eighty-eight pounds. Your body makes it and uses it up that fast.

The ATM of Energy

When your power plants are working well, you make plenty. You feel sharp, strong, and energized. When they're not, you run low. And running low on ATP is not like running low on gas, where you get a little warning and then stop. It's more like a brownout, everything works, but worse.

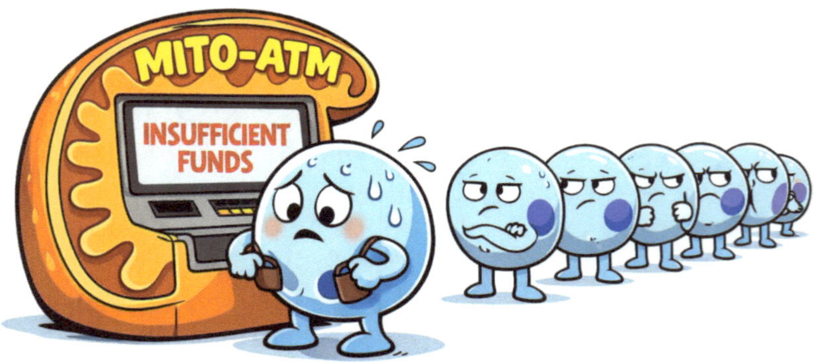

Every blink every heartbeat every thought costs ATP.
What happens when you run out?

You can still think, but not clearly. You can still exercise, but you're exhausted. You can still fight off a cold, but it takes two weeks instead of three days. You can still burn fat, but your body would rather store it.

This is the state most adults are walking around in. Not sick. Just underpowered.

The Doctor Visit Problem

Here's the thing about your doctor. They are very good at one specific job. That job is finding out if something has gone very, very wrong.

Your annual checkup is basically a check to make sure you haven't crashed yet. Blood pressure? Check. Cholesterol? Check. Blood sugar? Check. The doctor looks at the results, nods, and says those magic words: "Everything looks normal."

And you think, "Then why do I feel like I'm running on a phone that's been at 12% battery since Tuesday?"

Because the tests your doctor runs are not checking the power plants. They're checking the walls of the building. They look fine. Meanwhile, in the basement, every generator is sputtering.

Doctor Visit

This is not your doctor's fault. Doctors are trained to find disease. But what you have isn't a disease. It's a performance

problem. And nobody in medicine is really trained to look for that.

That's what this book is for.

What This Book Is Going to Teach You This book is going to teach you three things:

1. Why your power plants are struggling. (It's not just aging. It's missing parts.) 2. How to fix them, in the right order. (There's a system. It's called UCOS.) 3. What happens when you do. (You'll feel like a different person in 90 days.) No medical degree required. No

complicated diets. No expensive equipment. Just an understanding of how your body actually works, told in a way that makes sense, and a simple plan to give your 37 trillion tiny computers what they've been missing.

Let's get started.

The Simple Version

- Your body is made of 37 trillion cells. Each one is a tiny computer.
- Each cell has power plants called mitochondria. They make all your energy.
- When the power plants slow down, everything slows down: brain, energy, mood, weight, immune system.
- Your doctor checks if you're sick. Nobody checks if your power plants are running well. This book teaches you how to check, and how to fix them.

Chapter 2

Your Power Plants Are Rusty

Your mitochondria do not break overnight. They slip a little each year, and they lose about ten percent of their output every decade. And because it happens so gradually, you just adapt. You drink more coffee. You go to bed earlier. You tell yourself this is just what getting older feels like.

It isn't. It's what running low on the things your power plants need feels like.

Here's the good news. A car engine needs specific things to work. Oil, coolant, spark plugs, fuel, and clean air. If any one of those is missing, the engine runs badly. But if you put them back, the engine runs better.

Your power plants are the same way.

The 5 Things Your Power Plants Need Think of your mitochondria like a car engine. They need five things to run well.

1. Fuel (the food you eat)

Your mitochondria burn glucose and fat for fuel. No food, no fuel, simple enough. But here's the catch: the wrong food gunks up the engine. Ultra-processed food is like putting bad gasoline in a luxury car. It technically burns, but not cleanly. More on that in Chapter 7.

2. Spark Plugs (CoQ10)

CoQ10, say it like "cue-ten", is a molecule your mitochondria need to actually generate energy from fuel. Think of it like the spark plugs in your car engine. Without spark plugs, you can have a full tank of gas and the engine still won't fire right.

Here's a problem nobody tells you about. Your body makes CoQ10 on its own. But production drops as you age. And if you take a cholesterol drug called a statin, it drops even faster. Statins block the same pathway your body uses to make CoQ10. So you lower your cholesterol, and accidentally yank out your spark plugs.

If you're on a statin and you're tired all the time, this is worth looking into.

The Neglected Engine

3. Oil (magnesium)

Magnesium is the oil your power plants run on. And almost nobody has enough of it.

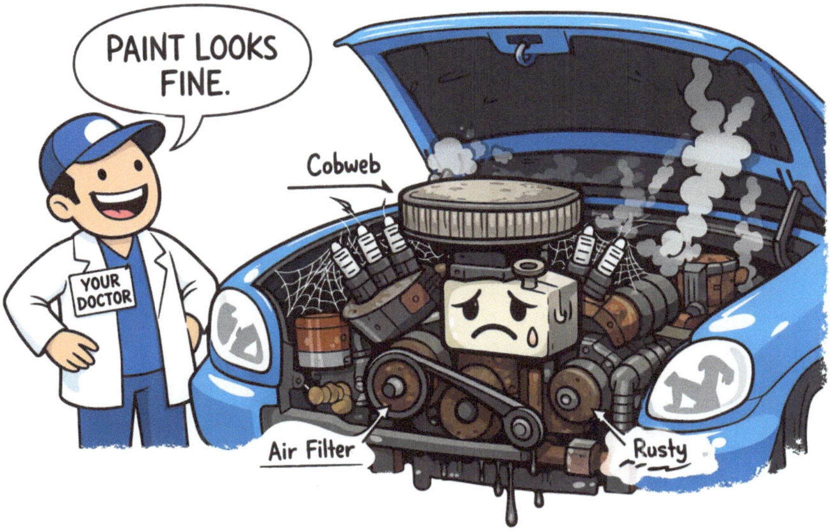

Here's the thing about magnesium that will blow your mind a little. Your energy molecule, ATP, can't actually work without magnesium attached to it. Scientists call the active form "Mg-ATP." Magnesium is not optional. It's not a nice extra. Without it, your ATP just sits there, useless.

It's like having a full tank of gas, good spark plugs, and a completely seized engine.

Over 300 chemical reactions in your body require magnesium to work. Three hundred. Sleep, blood sugar, muscle function, heart rhythm, nerve signals, all of them need magnesium. And nearly half of all Americans don't get enough.

4. Coolant (antioxidants)

When your power plants make energy, they also produce exhaust. That exhaust is called reactive oxygen species, which is a fancy way of saying "tiny sparks that damage things." Your antioxidants, like vitamins C and E, are the coolant system. They put out those sparks before they burn a hole in something.

When your antioxidant system is overwhelmed, those sparks start damaging your mitochondria themselves. Over time, this creates a vicious cycle: damaged power plants make more sparks, which causes more damage.

5. Clean Air (oxygen delivery)

Your mitochondria need oxygen to burn fuel. That oxygen comes from your blood. If your red blood cells can't carry oxygen well, or if your blood isn't flowing well, your power plants suffocate a little bit every day.

This is why exercise matters so much. More on that in Chapter 6. For now, just know that good oxygen delivery is step five.

The Slow Slide Nobody Notices Here's what happens to your power plants over time.

After age 30, you lose about 10% of your mitochondrial function per decade. Not all at once. Just slowly, quietly, steadily.

By 40, you're at about 90%. You notice you need a little more coffee.

By 50, you're at about 75%. You need that coffee earlier. You're tired by 3pm. Recovery after exercise takes longer.

By 60, you're at about 55%, running on just over half power. You say things like "I just don't have the energy I used to." And people nod like this is inevitable.

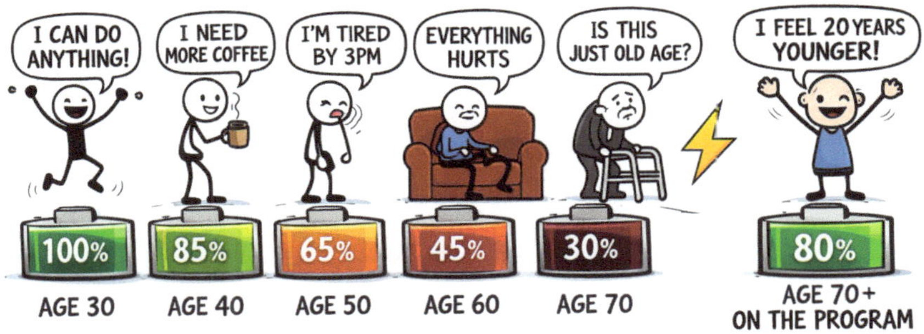
I CAN DO ANYTHING!
I NEED MORE COFFEE
I'M TIRED BY 3PM
EVERYTHING HURTS
IS THIS JUST OLD AGE?
I FEEL 20 YEARS YOUNGER!
100%
85%
65%
45%
30%
80%
AGE 30
AGE 40
AGE 50
AGE 60
AGE 70
AGE 70+ ON THE PROGRAM

It's not inevitable. It's a maintenance problem.

The 10% Per Decade Slide

Think about a car you love. You use it every day. You never change the oil. You never replace the spark plugs. You never flush the coolant. After a few years, it still runs, but not well. It hesitates before it starts. It gets worse gas mileage. It vibrates at highway speed. You tell yourself, "It's just getting old."

But an old car that's been maintained runs beautifully. A young car that's been ignored runs like junk.

Your mitochondria are the same.

The Test Your Doctor Isn't Running When most doctors check your magnesium, they run a serum magnesium test. They check how much magnesium is floating around in your blood.

This test is almost useless. And here's why.

Your body works very hard to keep your blood magnesium stable. Even if your cells are starving for magnesium, your body will pull it from your bones and your tissues to keep the blood level normal. So your blood looks fine. Meanwhile, your cells are empty.

It's like checking the water level in a reservoir by looking at the drinking fountain. The fountain might still be flowing. But the reservoir is nearly dry.

The test you want is called an RBC magnesium test, that's "red blood cell magnesium." This test looks inside the cells themselves. And when you run that test, a lot of people who "look fine" on regular labs turn out to be significantly depleted.

This matters because magnesium isn't just about energy. Low magnesium also causes muscle cramps. Poor sleep. Racing heart. Anxiety. Constipation. Migraines. High blood pressure. All things that doctors will treat with separate medications, when the real issue might be that the oil is low.

Magnesium: The Thing Nobody Checks

What to Do About It The good news: this stuff is fixable.

Adding CoQ10 back in is straightforward. Adding magnesium, specifically magnesium glycinate, which absorbs well and doesn't cause stomach issues, is one of the highest-return things you can do for your energy, sleep, and mood.

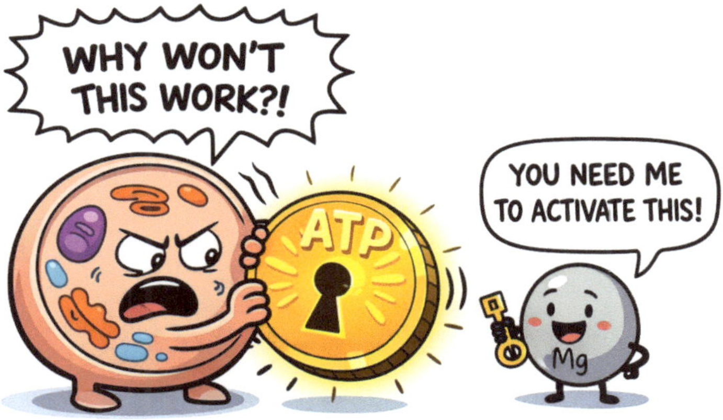
WHY WON'T THIS WORK?!
YOU NEED ME TO ACTIVATE THIS!
ATP
Mg

ATP without magnesium is like a car with a full tank but no key.

Getting your antioxidant status up through real food and targeted supplements puts out the sparks.

And fixing your oxygen delivery? That's exercise. Specifically, the kind of steady walking that gets your heart moving without making you want to die. We'll get into that in detail later.

The point of this chapter is simple. Your power plants are not getting old. They are getting neglected. And neglect is something you can fix.

The Simple Version

- Your power plants need 5 things: fuel, spark plugs (CoQ10), oil (magnesium), coolant (antioxidants), and clean air (oxygen).
- You lose about 10% of your mitochondrial power every decade after age 30. That's not aging, that's a maintenance problem.
- The magnesium test your doctor runs is nearly useless. Ask for an RBC magnesium test.

- Most of what you're blaming on "getting older" is actually a power plant that's low on parts.

Chapter 3

Zombie Cells and the Garbage Truck

Inside every cell there is a cleanup crew that hauls off broken parts. When that crew quits, the cell ends up like a car nobody services anymore, with the engine seizing and the owner still parking it in the garage all day.

Inside every cell, your body runs a continuous cleanup operation. It finds broken parts, worn-out machinery, and damaged mitochondria. It wraps them up, hauls them away, and recycles the raw materials into new, working parts. This process is called autophagy. Say it like this: aw-TAH-fuh-jee.

Autophagy literally means "self-eating." Which sounds horrifying. But it's actually the most important cleanup system you have. It's your cell's garbage truck, janitor, and recycling center all in one.

Here's the problem.

The garbage truck only runs when it's given the chance to run. And most people never give it that chance.

When Does the Garbage Truck Run? Your cleanup system has an on-switch and an off-switch.

The off-switch is: eating. Every time you eat, especially carbohydrates and protein, your body shifts into growth mode. It's busy processing food, storing energy, and building things. There's no time for cleanup.

The on-switch is: not eating. When your body runs low on incoming fuel, it flips into cleanup mode. It starts sorting through the junk and recycling what it can.

This is supposed to happen naturally, overnight, when you're sleeping and not eating. But here's what most people actually do.

They eat breakfast at 7am. They snack through the morning. They eat lunch. They have an afternoon snack. Dinner at 6pm. Then a bowl of cereal at 10pm before bed. They're asleep by 11pm and awake by 6am.

That's 15 hours of eating and only 8 hours of fasting. The garbage truck barely has time to warm up before you're shoveling more food in.

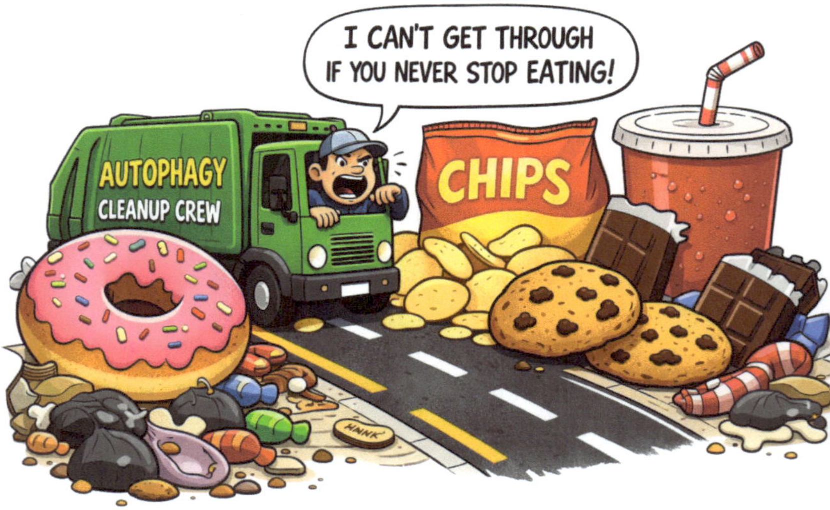
I CAN'T GET THROUGH IF YOU NEVER STOP EATING!
AUTOPHAGY
CLEANUP CREW
CHIPS

The Garbage Truck

The result? Garbage piles up. Broken cell parts accumulate. Damaged mitochondria stay in service instead of getting recycled. Over months and years, this slows everything down.

Imagine a restaurant kitchen that never gets cleaned. The cooks keep working, but the grease builds up, old food scraps pile in the corners, the equipment gets crusted and sticky. The food that comes out gets worse and worse. The kitchen isn't broken, it just hasn't been cleaned in years.

That's your cells without autophagy.

Zombie Cells: The Neighbors Who Won't Leave Now let's talk about something worse than piled-up garbage.

Some cells in your body get old and damaged to the point where they should die. Dying is actually the healthy thing for a cell to do when it's worn out. The body replaces old cells with new ones constantly. Your gut lining replaces itself every few days. Your red blood cells live about 120 days, then get recycled.

But some cells get stuck. They don't die. They don't work anymore either. They just sit there, broken, useless, and angry.

Scientists call these senescent cells. Say it like this: SEE-neh-sent. In this book, we're calling them what they are: zombie cells.

Zombie cells are a problem. A big problem.

Here's why. A healthy cell, when it dies, does it quietly. It packages itself up neatly and signals to the cleanup crew. Smooth, orderly, no mess.

A zombie cell won't do this. It just sits there and leaks. It pumps out inflammatory chemicals, little chemical signals that say "I'M IN TROUBLE" over and over. These chemicals irritate the neighboring cells. They cause the surrounding tissue to inflame. They make nearby cells more likely to become zombies themselves.

It's like having one neighbor who never throws out their trash. Their rotting garbage starts to smell. It attracts pests. It drives down property values for everyone on the block. And no matter how nicely you ask, they will not clean up.

Zombie Cells

The slow fire that zombie cells cause is called inflammaging, chronic, low-grade inflammation that builds up as you age. You can't feel it directly. There's no fever, no obvious swelling. But it's there, quietly making everything work a little worse.

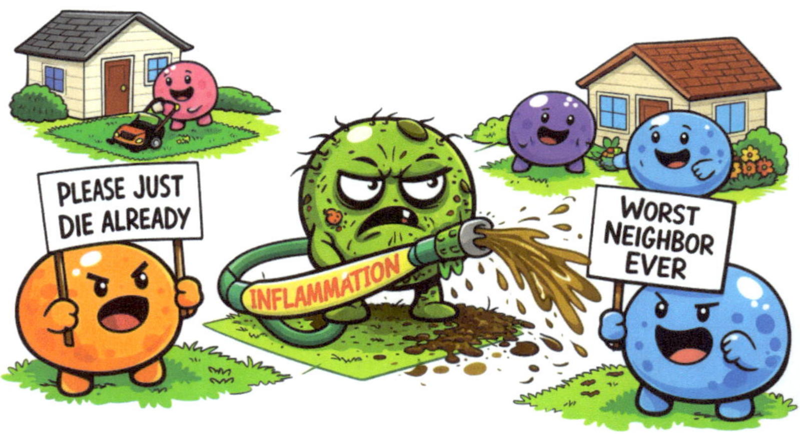

Senescent cells – they won't leave and they make everyone around them miserable.

Inflammaging is linked to almost every condition that gets worse with age. Heart disease. Diabetes. Alzheimer's. Arthritis. Even depression. Not because these conditions cause inflammation, but because inflammation creates the conditions where these problems thrive.

Turning On the Cleanup Crew

The good news is that you have real tools for this.

Fasting turns on the garbage truck. You don't need to fast for three days. A 12-to-14-hour overnight window, say, no eating after 7pm and not eating again until 7 or 8am, is enough to kick autophagy into gear. This isn't a diet. It's just giving your cleanup system the quiet time it needs.

Spermidine helps trigger autophagy. Spermidine (SPER-mih-deen) is a compound found naturally in foods like wheat germ, mushrooms, and aged cheese. It's one of the most powerful autophagy-triggering substances we know of. Your body makes less of it as you age, which is part of why cleanup slows down over time. Supplementing spermidine can turn on the garbage truck even when you're not fasting.

Fisetin and quercetin are zombie cell killers. These are compounds from plants, fisetin (FIZ-eh-tin) is found in strawberries; quercetin (KWER-seh-tin) is in onions and apples. They're called senolytics (see-no-LIT-iks), which means they help clear out those zombie cells. They don't just clean up the garbage. They evict the neighbor who won't leave.

The On/Off Switch

The Eating-All-Day Problem Here's something worth sitting with.

In human history, people have almost never had access to food 24 hours a day. For most of our existence, we ate when food was available and didn't eat when it wasn't. Our bodies evolved to be very good at cycling between eating and not eating.

In the last 50 years or so, constant food became available to most people in developed countries. We responded by eating constantly. And our bodies, which were never designed for this, started skipping the cleanup step.

You were designed to eat, then clean. Eat, then clean. Over and over, in a rhythm.

When you eat all day, you only do the first half of the cycle. The cleanup never happens.

This doesn't mean you need to suffer. It doesn't mean you need to feel hungry all the time or give up food you love. It just means giving your body a few hours a day to do the maintenance work it was designed to do.

Start with 12 hours. If you finish dinner by 7pm, don't eat again until 7am. That's it. The garbage truck needs that much time, at minimum, to get out of the garage and do its route.

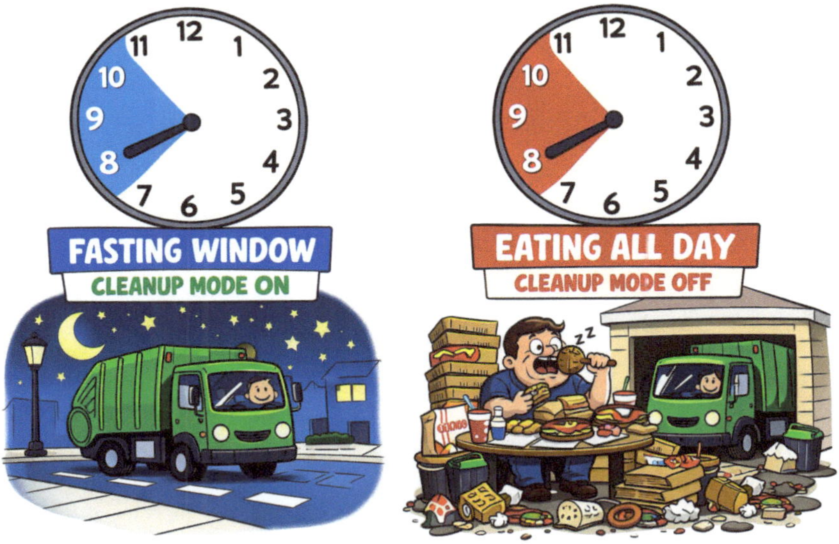

Your cells will thank you.

The Simple Version

- Autophagy is your body's garbage truck, it picks up broken parts and recycles them. It only runs when you're not eating.
- Zombie cells (senescent cells) won't die and won't work. They just leak inflammatory chemicals onto their neighbors.
- Eating all day keeps the garbage truck parked. A 12-14 hour overnight fast lets it run.
- Spermidine triggers cleanup even when you're not fasting. Fisetin and quercetin help clear out zombie cells.

Chapter 4

Your Body Has Two Modes (And You're Stuck in One)

Your body has the most sophisticated transmission ever created, and right now, it's stuck in the wrong gear.

You have exactly two operating modes. One is for building. One is for cleaning. They are supposed to take turns. Most Americans stopped letting them take turns about 50 years ago. And the consequences are now sitting around our waistlines and showing up in our brain fog.

Let's talk about the two modes.

Mode 1: Build Mode Your body has a switch called mTOR. Say it like: em-TOR. It stands for "mechanistic target of rapamycin," which is a mouthful that nobody needs to remember. Just call it the growth switch.

When mTOR is on, your body is in build mode. It builds muscle. It stores fat. It grows things. It makes copies of cells.

mTOR turns on when you eat protein. It turns on when you eat sugar. It turns on when your blood sugar spikes. It also turns on when you just sit still, because your body interprets sitting as "we must be resting and storing up for something."

Build mode is great. You need it. You need to build muscle. You need to store some energy. You need cells to copy themselves. mTOR is not bad.

It's just not supposed to be on all the time.

Mode 2: Cleanup Mode Your other switch is called AMPK. Say it like: A-M-P-K. Think of it as the cleanup switch.

When AMPK is on, your body is in cleanup mode. It burns stored fat for fuel. It triggers autophagy, the garbage truck from Chapter 3. It recycles old, broken parts. It repairs damaged cells. It does all the maintenance work your body needs to stay sharp and functional.

AMPK turns on when you run low on fuel, when you're fasting, or exercising, or when your blood sugar drops. It's your body's way of saying, "Okay, no new food coming in. Time to clean house and burn what we've got stored."

Here's the key thing about these two switches.

They are a seesaw. When one is up, the other is down. When mTOR is fully on, build mode, AMPK can't run. Cleanup is off. And when AMPK is fully on, cleanup mode, mTOR is suppressed. Building slows.

The Seesaw

Your body was designed to alternate. Eat a meal, mTOR goes up, AMPK goes down. Build for a few hours. Then stop eating, AMPK goes up, mTOR goes down. Clean for several hours. Eat again. Clean again. Repeat forever.

That rhythm is what keeps you healthy.

How We Broke the Seesaw Here's what modern life did to that rhythm.

The average American eats for about 15 to 16 hours a day. Breakfast at 7am. Snack at 10. Lunch at noon. Snack at 3. Dinner at 7. Evening snack before bed at 10pm.

Every time you eat, every single time, mTOR spikes. Build mode turns on. AMPK gets pushed down. Cleanup stops.

At 15 hours of eating per day, AMPK barely gets a window to work at all.

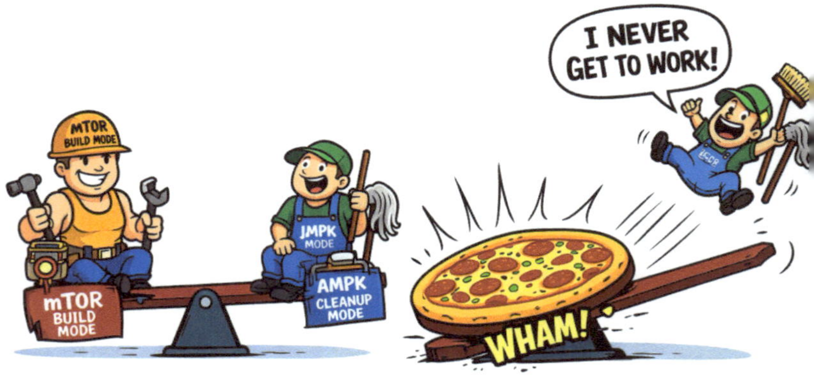

And then we add the sitting. The average American sits for 9 to 10 hours a day. Sitting keeps blood sugar elevated. It keeps mTOR elevated. It keeps AMPK suppressed. More build mode. Less cleanup.

Stuck in Build Mode

The result is what scientists call "deregulated nutrient sensing." In plain English: your body's build-vs-clean system got stuck in one position. Always building. Never cleaning.

Think about a city that's always under construction. New condos going up everywhere. But the old, condemned buildings from

1970 are still standing. Nobody has knocked them down. New construction keeps going up right next to crumbling, toxic, half-collapsed buildings.

That's your body when mTOR never turns off. New fat cells going up right next to old zombie cells. New inflammation building on top of old inflammation.

You grow, mostly wider.

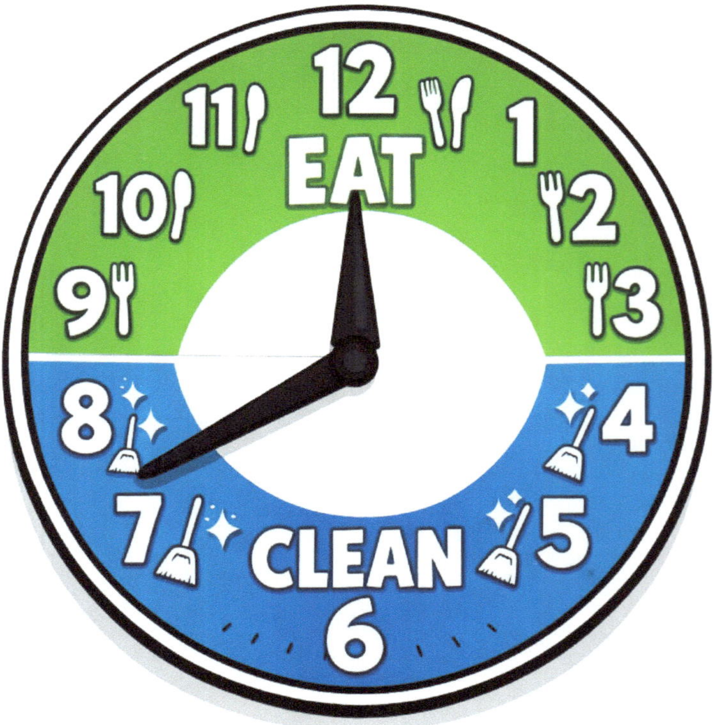

Your body was designed to **eat then clean.**

Eat then clean.

We broke the cycle by eating all day.
Fix this one thing and you fix half
the problems in this book.

How to Fix the Seesaw The fix is not complicated. But it requires actually doing something different.

Time-restricted eating. Pick an 8-to-10-hour window during the day when you eat. Outside that window, you don't eat. This gives AMPK a real chance to run.

If you eat your first meal at 9am and your last meal at 7pm, that's a 10-hour eating window. You've given your body 14 hours of cleanup time overnight. This is not a diet. You're not eating less food, you're just moving it into a shorter window. For most people, this alone makes a meaningful difference in energy, fat loss, and brain clarity.

Zone 2 exercise. Zone 2 is a specific level of effort, hard enough that your heart is working and you're breathing faster than normal, but easy enough that you could hold a conversation. You can talk. You just don't particularly want to.

At Zone 2 intensity, your body burns fat for fuel. This triggers AMPK. It activates the cleanup switch. It tells your cells to start clearing junk and recycling old parts.

You don't have to run. You don't have to kill yourself at the gym. A brisk walk, the kind where you're moving with purpose and your breath is slightly elevated, is Zone 2. Walking is one of the most powerful things you can do for your cells.

Zone 2 also does something remarkable. It signals your body to build new mitochondria. More power plants. We'll talk more about that in Chapter 6.

Resistance training. This is the other half of exercise. Two sessions a week of lifting weights, or any form of resistance training, tells your body to build and maintain muscle. Muscle is not just for looking strong. Muscle is one of the most metabolically active tissues in your body. More muscle means better blood sugar control, better hormones, better everything.

This Is Not a Diet Let's be very clear about something.

This is not a diet. There is no list of forbidden foods. There is no calorie counting. There is no suffering required.

This is about rhythm.

Your body was built to cycle between building and cleaning. Your ancestors did it without thinking about it, because food wasn't available 24 hours a day. You have to be a little more deliberate about it, because you live in a world with a 7-Eleven on every corner.

But the biology is simple. Give your body a window to clean. Move enough to trigger the cleanup switch. Your cells will do the rest.

They've been waiting for the chance.

The Simple Version

• Your body has two modes: mTOR (build) and AMPK (clean). They are a seesaw, when one is up, the other is down.

• Eating all day keeps mTOR stuck on and never lets AMPK do its job. Your body builds and stores but never cleans.

• Fix it with a simple eating window (eat in 8-10 hours, fast overnight) and Zone 2 exercise (a brisk walk where you can talk but don't want to).

• This is not a diet. It's letting your body do what it was designed to do.

Chapter 5

Sleep: When the Repair Crew Comes Out

You know how cities fix the roads at 2am when nobody's driving? That's sleep. Your body is doing construction, hauling waste, and filling potholes, but only if you're actually asleep.

Most people think sleep is passive. You close your eyes, you stop doing things, you wake up. Not much is happening in the meantime.

This is completely wrong.

Sleep is the most metabolically active period of your day. Your brain is firing intensely. Your body is making hormones. Your cells are breaking down damaged parts and building new ones. Your immune system is processing information. Your memories are being filed.

And most importantly, your power plants are being repaired.

Shortcut sleep, or get bad quality sleep, and you skip the repair window. Do it often enough, and the damage starts to compound.

The Repair Crew When you fall into deep sleep, the kind called slow-wave sleep, or stages 3 and 4, something remarkable happens. Your body releases a surge of growth hormone.

Growth hormone isn't just for teenagers who want to get taller. In adults, growth hormone is the signal that tells your body to repair everything. Muscles that got tiny tears from exercise get rebuilt. Bone tissue gets strengthened. Organ cells that are worn out get replaced. Mitochondria that are damaged get broken down and recycled.

This is when the repair crew comes out.

And here's the thing about growth hormone: it peaks during the first few hours of deep sleep. If you go to bed at midnight and wake up at 5am, you're cutting the repair shift short. The crew barely gets started before you're telling them to pack up and go home.

Night Shift

Think about how road construction works. Cities can't repair the main roads during the day. Too much traffic. So the repair crews come out at 2am, when the streets are empty. They repave, they

patch potholes, they fix the drainage. By 6am, the crews are gone and the road is smooth.

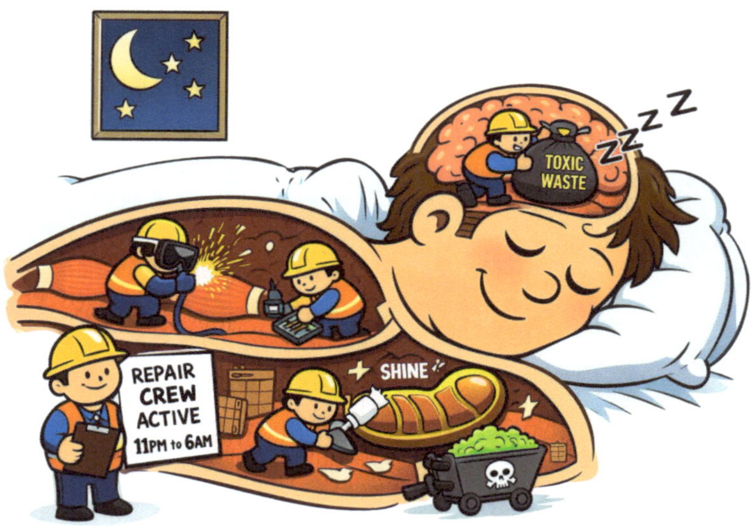

Your body works the same way. The repair crews come out when traffic is low, when you're deeply asleep and your systems are quiet. If you never give them that window, the potholes just get bigger. Eventually the road starts to fall apart.

Your Brain Gets Washed Here's something that was only discovered in 2012, and it's one of the most astonishing things in modern biology.

Your brain has its own cleaning system. It's called the glymphatic system. Say it like: glie-FAT-ic.

During sleep, your brain cells actually shrink slightly. This opens up tiny channels between them. Fluid, essentially a special kind of spinal fluid, flows through those channels and washes the brain.

What does it wash out? Toxic waste. Including a protein called beta-amyloid. Say it like: bay-ta AM-ih-loyd.

Beta-amyloid is one of the main substances that builds up in the brains of people with Alzheimer's disease. It's a sticky, clumping protein that gums up the brain's communication pathways over time.

Your glymphatic system is supposed to wash it out every single night. But the glymphatic system only really runs during deep sleep.

Skip sleep, and the brain wash doesn't happen. The beta-amyloid builds up a little bit more each night. Over years and decades, this adds up. It's one of the reasons chronic poor sleep is a major risk factor for Alzheimer's disease.

The Brain Wash

You have a brain car wash. It only runs when you're asleep. Every night you sleep well, it runs its cycle. Every night you don't, whether because you didn't sleep long enough, or your sleep was broken, or you had three drinks before bed, the wash is partial or skipped entirely.

This is not scare tactics. This is just biology. And it's very fixable.

Melatonin: Not What You Think It Is When people hear the word melatonin, they think "sleep pill." Go to CVS, grab a 10mg tablet, take it, pass out.

But melatonin is not primarily a sedative. That's not its main job.

Melatonin is a signaling hormone. Its first job is to tell your body that it's nighttime and to start winding down. Dim the lights on

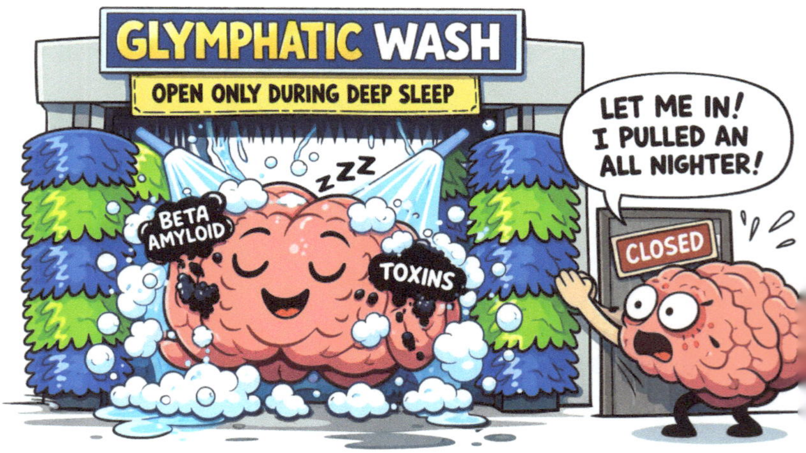
GLYMPHATIC WASH
OPEN ONLY DURING DEEP SLEEP
ZZZ
BETA AMYLOID
TOXINS
LET ME IN! I PULLED AN ALL NIGHTER!
CLOSED

the organs. Slow the heart rate a bit. Lower the body temperature slightly. Signal the repair crews to get ready.

But here's what most people don't know. Melatonin is also one of the most powerful antioxidants in your body. Specifically, it protects your mitochondria overnight. Remember the coolant system from Chapter

2, the antioxidants that put out the sparks your power plants create? Melatonin is a major part of that system.

While you sleep, your mitochondria are doing heavy repair work. This generates a lot of those reactive sparks. Melatonin helps neutralize them before they cause further damage. In this way, melatonin is not just helping you sleep, it's actively protecting your power plants during the most intense repair shift of the day.

Now, here's the problem with that 10mg CVS horse pill.

Your body makes melatonin naturally, and in much smaller amounts than you'd find in those over-the-counter pills. The right physiological dose, the one that signals your body correctly without overwhelming it, is somewhere around 300 to 600 micrograms. That's 0.3 to 0.6 milligrams.

The standard CVS gummy? 5 to 10 milligrams. That's 15 to 30 times more than your body uses naturally.

A huge dose of melatonin doesn't give you better sleep. It just knocks you out, often without giving you the deep, restorative sleep stages you actually need. And over time, your brain can stop producing its own melatonin in normal amounts, because you've been supplying it so aggressively from the outside.

Melatonin: CVS vs. Reality

The right approach is low-dose melatonin, 600 micrograms (0.6mg), taken about 30 to 60 minutes before bed. This mimics what your body does naturally. It tells your systems to wind down. It protects your mitochondria. And it supports the deep sleep stages where the real repair happens.

The Sleep Stack That Works Good sleep is not just about one thing. It's a system. Here are the pieces that matter most.

GABA (50mg). GABA is the main calming neurotransmitter in your brain, say it like "gamma-aminobutyric acid," or just "GABA." It's the brake pedal for your nervous system. When you're anxious, overthinking, or wired at bedtime, your GABA is low and your excitatory neurotransmitters are winning the argument.

A low dose of GABA taken before bed, 50 milligrams, not the big doses you sometimes see, helps your brain shift from "processing the day" mode to "winding down" mode. It doesn't knock you out. It just eases the mental chatter so you can actually fall asleep.

Melatonin (600mcg). As above. Low dose, physiological, protective.

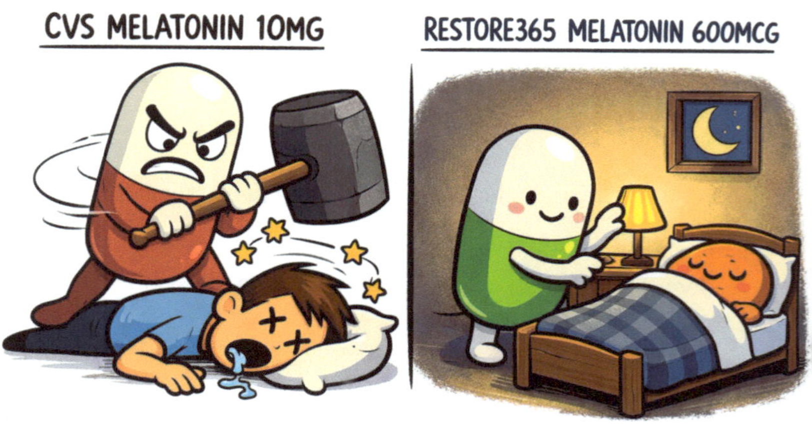

More is not better. The right dose helps.

Magnesium glycinate. Remember magnesium from Chapter 2, your power plants' oil? Magnesium also relaxes muscles and calms the nervous system. Magnesium glycinate, "glycinate" refers to how it's attached to an amino acid that helps it absorb, is the form that gets into the brain most easily. It helps your muscles release tension, calms mental restlessness, and supports deep sleep architecture.

These three together, low-dose GABA, physiological melatonin, and magnesium glycinate, support the specific sleep stages where your body does its most important repair work. Not by knocking you out. By giving your nervous system what it needs to wind down naturally and sleep deeply.

Why This Matters More Than You Think Bad sleep is not just "feeling groggy in the morning." This is what happens inside your cells when you consistently get poor sleep.

Growth hormone drops. Your repair crews are understaffed and undertrained. Muscles don't recover. Organs don't get maintained. Mitochondria don't get recycled.

The brain wash runs poorly. Beta-amyloid and other waste products accumulate. Cognition slips. Memory gets worse. Over years, the risk of neurodegenerative disease climbs.

Your mitochondria don't get antioxidant protection through the night. They take more damage. They run less efficiently. Your energy gets worse.

Cortisol, your stress hormone, rises when you don't sleep enough. High cortisol tells your body to store fat, especially belly fat. It suppresses testosterone. It suppresses your immune system. It keeps mTOR elevated, which means your cleanup mode (AMPK) gets further suppressed.

One bad night is recoverable. Chronic poor sleep, night after night of 5 or 6 hours, or sleep that never reaches the deep stages, is not something you can just power through. It quietly erodes your systems until you feel exactly like the person in Chapter 1: not sick, just running on 60% power.

The repair crew needs a full shift. Give it to them.

A Few Simple Rules for Better Sleep You don't need a $4,000 mattress. You need the right environment and the right timing.

Keep it dark. Even small amounts of light during sleep, a phone screen, a streetlight through the curtains, the little LED on your TV, suppresses melatonin and disrupts sleep stages. Blackout curtains or a sleep mask make a real difference.

Keep it cool. Your body needs to drop its core temperature slightly to initiate and maintain deep sleep. A room around 65-68°F is ideal for most people. If you wake up sweaty, your room is too warm.

Stop eating 2-3 hours before bed. Digestion raises your core body temperature and keeps mTOR elevated. Both of these fight deep sleep. Finishing dinner by 7pm if you're going to bed at 10pm gives your body a chance to cool down and shift modes.

No alcohol before bed. Alcohol makes you feel sleepy but fragments your sleep architecture. You fall asleep quickly and then spend the rest of the night in light, non-restorative stages. Your brain wash barely runs. Your repair crew barely works.

Consistent wake time. Your body's circadian rhythm, its internal clock, is anchored most strongly by what time you wake up, not what time you go to bed. Pick a wake time and stick to it every day, including weekends. This does more for sleep quality than almost anything else.

The road crew comes out every night. Your only job is to clear the roads and stay out of their way.

The Simple Version

- Sleep is when your body repairs itself. Growth hormone peaks during deep sleep and tells your cells to rebuild.
- Your brain has a car wash (the glymphatic system) that only runs during deep sleep. It flushes out toxic proteins linked to Alzheimer's.
- Melatonin is not just a sleep pill, it's an antioxidant that protects your mitochondria overnight. Use the low dose (600mcg), not the CVS sledgehammer version.
- GABA, low-dose melatonin, and magnesium glycinate together support the deep sleep stages where the real repair happens.

Chapter 6

Exercise: The Only Thing That Does Everything

There is one intervention that improves every system in your body at the same time. Not the supplement on the counter. Not that expensive IV drip you've been reading about. Only exercise.

Let that sink in for a second. You have a free, always-available tool that builds new mitochondria (my-toe-CON-dree-uh, your cell's power plants) and removes the damaged ones at the same time. And most people skip it because they'd rather watch one more episode of something.

We're going to fix that. Starting with understanding what exercise actually does inside your cells.

What Happens When You Walk Fast There's a specific kind of exercise called Zone 2. Here's the simple definition: you're moving fast enough that you could talk,

but you really don't want to. A brisk walk. A comfortable jog. A bike ride where you're breathing a little harder than normal.

That level of effort, not too easy, not too hard, does something amazing inside your cells.

It flips a switch called PGC-1 alpha (just say "PGC-one-alpha", or just say "the build switch"). This switch tells your cells to build new power plants. This process has a big name: mitochondrial biogenesis (by-oh-JEN-eh-sis). It means "making new mitochondria."

Your body literally manufactures new power plants when you move at a sustained, moderate pace. More power plants means more energy. More energy means sharper brain, better mood, faster metabolism, more fat burning, all day long.

If Exercise Were a Pill

But wait. There's more.

The Cleanup Crew Shows Up Too At the same time Zone 2 exercise triggers new power plant construction, it also triggers something called mitophagy (MY-toe-fay-jee). "Mito" = power plant. "Phagy" = eating. Mitophagy is your body's way of finding the old, rusty, broken power plants and recycling them.

Think about that for a second.

One single walk builds the new and demolishes the old. At the same time.

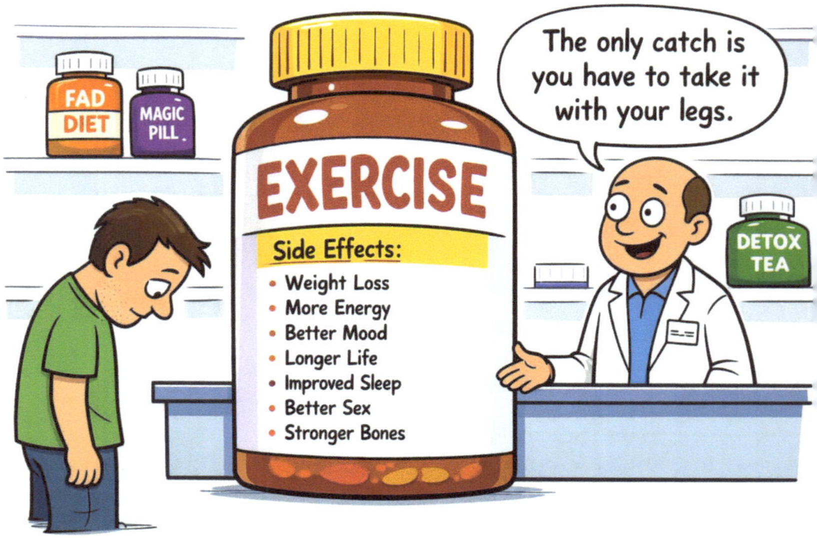
The only catch is you have to take it with your legs.
FAD DIET
MAGIC PILL
EXERCISE
Side Effects:
Weight Loss
More Energy
Better Mood
Longer Life
Improved Sleep
Better Sex
Stronger Bones
DETOX TEA

In Chapter 3, you learned about autophagy, your body's garbage truck that cleans up broken cell parts. Mitophagy is that same garbage truck, but specifically for your power plants. And the key trigger for that garbage truck showing up is sustained aerobic movement.

No movement. No garbage truck. Broken power plants pile up. Energy output drops. Everything gets worse.

This is why exercise is not optional. This is not about looking good at the beach. This is about whether your 37 trillion cells have working power plants or not.

The Two-for-One

The Second Kind: Resistance Training Zone 2 builds and cleans your power plants. But there's a second type of exercise you also need, resistance training.

That means lifting weights, doing bodyweight exercises, using resistance bands, or anything that makes your muscles push or pull against a load.

Why? Because muscle is not just something that looks good in a tank top. Muscle is your body's metabolic engine. More muscle means:

• You burn more calories, even sitting still • Your hormones stay stronger longer (testosterone, growth hormone)

• Your blood sugar gets controlled more effectively • You get stronger, which matters a lot after age 40 When you lift weights, you flip a different switch, the mTOR switch. Remember mTOR from Chapter 4? It's the growth switch. In this context, that's a good thing. You're telling your muscles to grow. Testosterone and growth hormone respond. Your metabolism speeds up. Your bones get stronger.

Zone 2 is for your power plants. Resistance training is for your structure. You need both.

Zone 2 vs. Resistance Training

The Minimum Effective Dose Now, how much do you actually need?

Here's the honest answer: more than most people do. But less than you probably fear.

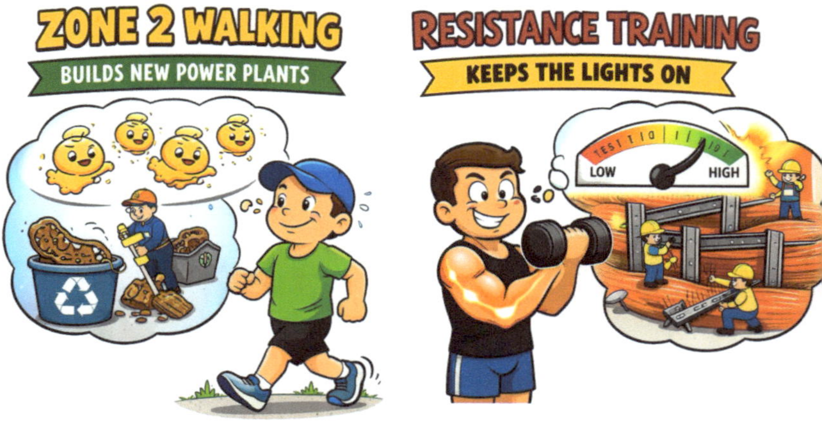

Walking builds new power plants. Lifting keeps the lights on. You need both.

The research-backed minimum for real results is:

• 150 minutes per week of Zone 2, that's just 30 minutes, five days a week, of walking fast enough that you can talk but don't want to • 2 resistance training sessions per week, 30 to 45 minutes each, working your major muscle groups That's it. That's the starting dose. You don't need a gym membership on day one. You need a good pair of shoes and a dumbbell or two.

If you're doing zero right now, start with 10 minutes. Walk for 10 minutes after dinner. That's the crack in the door. Every bit counts.

"I Don't Have Time" Let's do some math.

There are 168 hours in a week. The minimum dose of exercise requires about 4 of them.

You need 2.5 hours of Zone 2 walking. You need 1 to 1.5 hours of resistance training. Total: about 3.5 to 4 hours.

That leaves 164 hours for everything else.

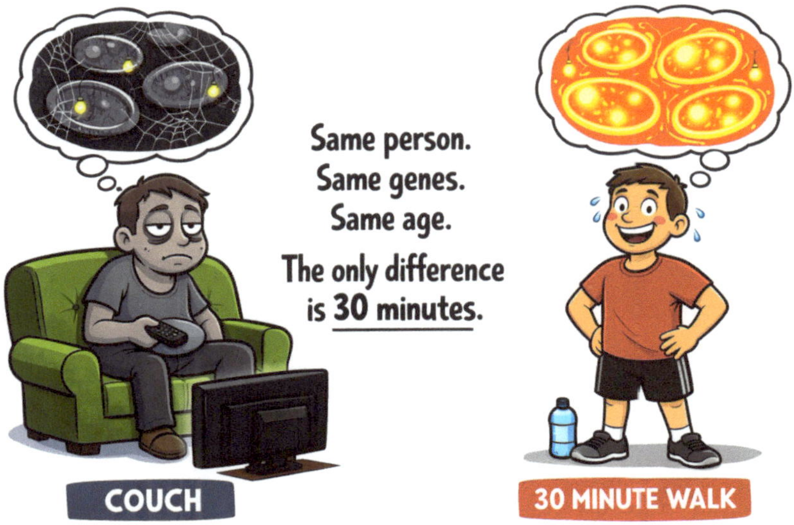
Same person.
Same genes.
Same age.
The only difference is 30 minutes.
COUCH
30 MINUTE WALK

The average American watches 27 hours of television per week. Exercise takes less than 15% of that.

This is not a time problem. It's a priority problem. And the reason to reprioritize isn't that your doctor told you to. It's that every chapter of this book links back to movement. Sleep quality

improves. Stress hormones drop. Blood sugar gets controlled. Brain fog clears. Power plants multiply.

Exercise is not a chapter in this story. It's the engine the whole story runs on.

No Pill Does This Here's something important to understand before we move on.

You can take NAD+ supplements. You can take CoQ10. You can take magnesium. You can get peptide injections. You can get an IV drip at a wellness clinic. All of these things can help. (And some of them are part of the plan in Chapters 9 and 10.)

But none of them, not one, triggers mitochondrial biogenesis the way Zone 2 exercise does. None of them triggers mitophagy the way Zone 2 does. The two signals that build new power plants and destroy old ones at the same time require physical movement to unlock.

You can supplement around the edges of what exercise does. You cannot replace it.

The good news? You don't need to become a marathon runner. You don't need to join CrossFit. You don't need to suffer. Zone 2 means comfortable. Sustainable. Something you can do every day without destroying yourself.

Start at 10 minutes. Work up to 30. Then 45. The power plants will follow.

The Simple Version

- Exercise is the only thing that builds new power plants (mitochondria) and removes broken ones at the same time. No pill does both.
- Zone 2 exercise, walking fast enough to talk but not want to, triggers both new growth and old cleanup. Do 150 minutes per week minimum.
- Resistance training (weights, bodyweight exercises) builds muscle, boosts testosterone and growth hormone, and speeds up your metabolism. Do it twice a week.
- This is not about looking good. It's about whether your 37 trillion cells have working power plants. Everything else in this book works better when you move.

Chapter 7

Food Is Fuel, Not Entertainment

There are over 43,000 stores in America whose entire business model is selling you sugar, and the healthy chains keep going out of business.

That is not a coincidence. That is a business plan. And your body is paying the bill.

Let's talk about food, what your cells actually need, why most Americans aren't getting it, and what the Sugar Nation has done to your brain, your hormones, and your energy levels without you noticing.

Your Cells Are a Construction Site Think about building a house. You need lumber, concrete, wiring, insulation, nails, plumbing. Actual building materials.

Now imagine a truck pulls up and dumps fifty thousand packing peanuts at the construction site. Colorful. Plentiful. But completely useless for building anything.

"There's plenty of material here," the driver says.

That's ultra-processed food. Calories. Lots of them. But almost none of the actual building materials your cells need to repair themselves, make new power plants, or keep your brain running.

Your cells need protein. Minerals. Vitamins. Healthy fats. Real things. Real materials. Without them, you can eat all day and still be running on fumes.

Building Materials vs. Packing Peanuts

The Ultra-Processed Problem Here's a number that should stop you cold: 60% of the average American's diet is ultra-processed food.

That means chips, cookies, fast food, frozen meals, sugary cereals, packaged snacks, and anything where the ingredient list reads like a chemistry exam.

These foods have been engineered to taste great and make you want more. They contain plenty of calories. But they've been

stripped of the micronutrients, magnesium, zinc, B vitamins, minerals, that your power plants actually need to function.

You're filling your gas tank. But you're not maintaining the engine. No oil. No spark plugs. No coolant.

And then you wonder why you're tired.

The Sugar Nation Now let's talk about the elephant in the room. Or rather, the 43,000 elephants.

Drive down any major street in any American city and count the businesses whose entire purpose is to sell sugar. Not restaurants that happen to serve dessert. Stores where sugar is the whole point.

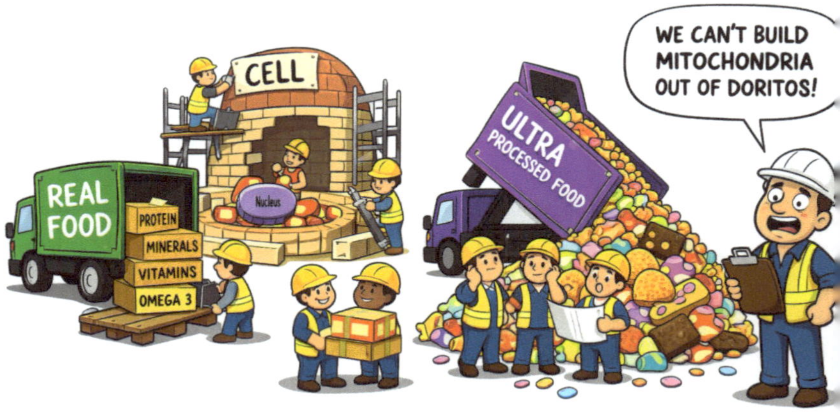

Swig. Crumbl. Dutch Bros. 7 Brew. Dunkin'. Starbucks. Insomnia Cookies. Nothing Bundt Cakes. Krispy Kreme. Cold Stone. Smoothie King. Jamba. Cinnabon.

The numbers are real. Add up just the major chains, dirty soda shops, cookie chains, doughnut shops, sugar-heavy coffee chains, ice cream stores, bubble tea shops, pretzel chains, and "healthy" smoothie shops that are anything but, and you get over 43,000 storefronts in the United States that exist primarily to sell sugar.

In a single year, 2025, 7 Brew opened 280 new stands, Crumbl added 81 stores, Dutch Bros added 170 locations, and Swig grew 54%. That's nearly 700 new sugar-delivery storefronts from just seven chains in one year.

While all of this was happening, Sweetgreen, the salad chain, lost $134 million and started closing locations. Veggie Grill closed 40% of its stores.

The market has spoken. And the market is making people sick.

The Sugar Strip Mall

How Much Sugar Are We Talking? The American Heart Association recommends no more than 25 grams of added sugar per day for women, and 37.5 grams per day for men.

Here's what's in some of your favorite spots:

- One Crumbl cookie: 60 to 80 grams of sugar
- One Swig dirty soda: 80 to 100 grams of sugar

• One Starbucks Venti Frappuccino: 67 to 102 grams of sugar (some seasonal flavors) One Crumbl cookie is three to four days' worth of recommended sugar. In one cookie.

The average American consumes about 300% of the daily recommended amount of added sugar. Every day.

And we wonder why we're tired. Why we're foggy. Why we're fat. Why we can't focus. Why our testosterone is in the basement.

There's a study called the Caronia study. It found that one single 75-gram glucose load, roughly the sugar in a large dirty soda, drops testosterone in men by 25%. Not a tiny bit. Twenty-five percent. And it stays low for two hours.

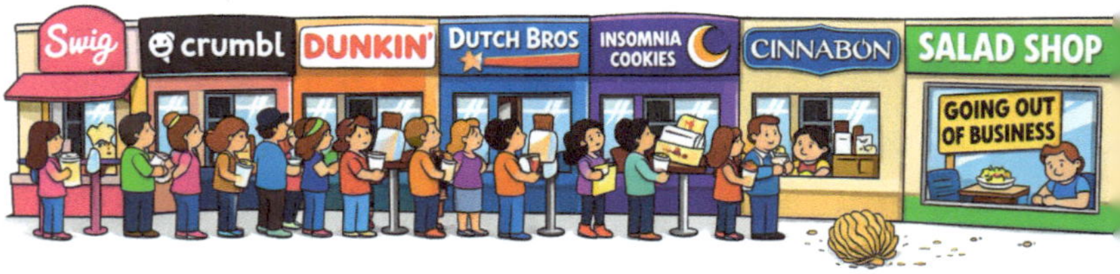

43,000 stores in America exist to sell sugar. This is not an accident. This is a business model.

If you're drinking a sugary drink every day, your testosterone is being robbed every single day. Nobody connects the dots. But now you can.

Sugar and Your Brain It's not just your hormones.

A 2024 analysis looked at 40 different studies covering 1.2 million people. What did it find? People with high sugar intake had a 21% increased risk of depression.

Sugar causes inflammation in your brain. It disrupts the signals your neurons use to communicate. It triggers blood sugar swings that leave you anxious, irritable, and foggy. And then, because misery loves company, the crash makes you crave more sugar.

This is not a willpower problem. It's a biochemistry problem. And it's being fed by 43,000 stores designed specifically to keep you coming back tomorrow.

Dr. Steve's Truth Bomb: Lettuce Is a Carb Here's something patients hear in the clinic that stops them cold.

"Doc, I barely eat any carbs. I have a big salad every day."

"What's in the salad?"

"Lettuce, tomatoes, cucumbers, a little dressing."

"Okay. Is lettuce a fat?"

"No."

"Is it a protein?"

"No."

"Then what is it?"

Silence. Then: "...a carb?"

Yes. Lettuce is a carb. A very good, very low-sugar, very high-fiber carb, but a carb. So is every vegetable. This isn't a reason to fear vegetables. Vegetables are some of the best food you can eat. But understanding that carbohydrates aren't just donuts and bread helps you see food more clearly.

Not all carbs are the same. A carrot and a Crumbl cookie are both technically carbs. Only one of them destroys your hormones and tanks your energy.

The Simple Rules You don't need a nutrition degree. You need two rules.

Rule 1: If it had a face, grew in dirt, or fell off a tree, eat it.

Chicken, beef, fish, eggs. Potatoes, carrots, broccoli, spinach. Apples, oranges, berries, bananas. These are real foods. Your cells know what to do with them. They've been doing it for millions of years.

Rule 2: If it came from a factory with ingredients you can't pronounce, eat less of it.

Not zero. Not never. Just less. A lot less.

Protein: The Building Block You're Probably Skipping Your cells rebuild themselves constantly. Every structure, every enzyme, every power plant, all made of protein.

The research-backed target is 1.6 to 2.0 grams of protein per kilogram of body weight, per day. For a 180-pound person (about 82 kg), that's roughly 130 to 164 grams of protein per day.

The easiest way to hit that? Put a palm-sized piece of protein at every meal. Chicken breast. Salmon. Eggs. Ground beef. Greek yogurt. A palm of protein. Every meal. Non-negotiable.

The Palm Rule

The Bottom Line Your cells are a construction crew. They show up every day ready to build, repair, and maintain. But they need real materials.

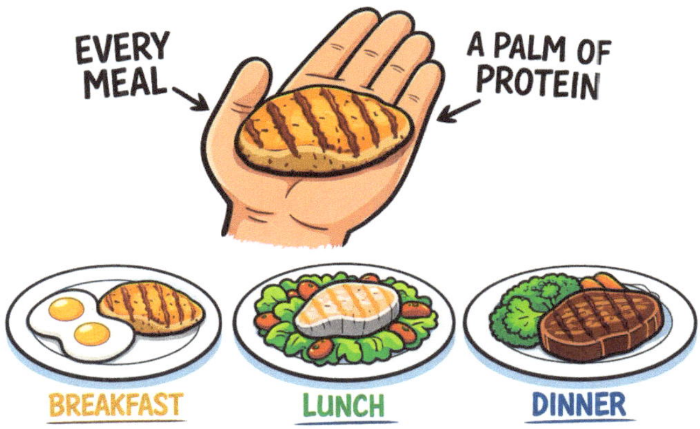

Every meal. A palm of protein.
Your cells need the building blocks. Give them the blocks.

Protein. Minerals. Vitamins. Real food.

What most Americans give them is colorful packaging, engineered flavors, and a sugar spike that crashes their hormones, inflames their brain, and empties their energy tank by 2pm.

You don't have to be perfect. But you do have to be honest about what you're actually feeding your 37 trillion power plants.

The Simple Version

- 60% of the average American diet is ultra-processed food. It has calories but almost none of the building materials your cells need.
- There are 43,000+ stores in America whose entire job is selling sugar. The average American eats 300% of the recommended daily amount. One Crumbl cookie is three days' worth.
- Sugar drops testosterone 25% per glucose load. It increases

depression risk by 21%. It's not in your head, it's in your biochemistry.

- Simple rules: put a palm of protein at every meal, eat real food (face, dirt, or tree), and eat a lot less of anything that came from a factory.

Chapter 8

Stress, Mood, and the Hormone Crash

But that's modern life. And your cells are paying the price.

The Bear Is Everywhere Your stress response is a marvel of engineering. A threat appears, a predator, a car swerving toward you, a very bad piece of news, and your brain sends a signal in about one-tenth of a second. Your heart speeds up. Blood pumps to your muscles. Your liver dumps sugar into your bloodstream for fast fuel. Your focus narrows to the threat.

This is called the fight-or-flight response. It works great. For two minutes.

Then the bear is gone. Your body stands down. Hormones reset. You go back to normal.

The problem is that modern life doesn't have a bear. It has a flood of bear-sized signals that never stop.

Emails at midnight. Bills. Traffic. A difficult boss. Conflict with a spouse. A news cycle designed to make you feel like the world is

ending. Your brain cannot tell the difference between "actual bear" and "work email about the quarterly report." To your nervous system, stress is stress.

So the alarm stays on. And on. And on.

What Chronic Stress Does to Your Cells When the fight-or-flight response fires, your adrenal glands (the little guys sitting on top of your kidneys) pump out a hormone called cortisol. Cortisol is your stress hormone. It's not bad. You need it. In the morning, cortisol naturally peaks to wake you up and get you moving.

The problem is what happens when it stays high all day, every day.

Chronically high cortisol tells your mitochondria, your power plants, to switch from "repair and rebuild" mode into "survive and conserve" mode.

In survival mode, your cells stop investing in the future. They stop repairing DNA. They stop building new power plants. They stop doing the slow, expensive work of maintenance. They just try to get through the day.

This is smart when you're actually running from a bear. It is disastrous when you're sitting at a desk feeling vaguely anxious about nothing in particular.

Over weeks and months, this shift wrecks your energy, your mood, your immune system, and your hormones.

Running from the Bear

What Sugar Does to Your Testosterone Here's a connection most people have never made, and it changes everything once you see it.

When you eat or drink sugar, your blood glucose spikes. Insulin floods in to manage it. And as part of that hormonal cascade, testosterone drops.

One study, the Caronia study, found that a single 75-gram glucose load dropped testosterone levels in men by 25%. Not eventually. Right then. Within two hours. The men's testosterone fell by a quarter from one sugary drink.

Now think about this: the average American dirty soda from Swig contains 80 to 100 grams of sugar. A Starbucks Frappuccino can hit 67 to 102 grams. One Crumbl cookie packs 60 to 80 grams.

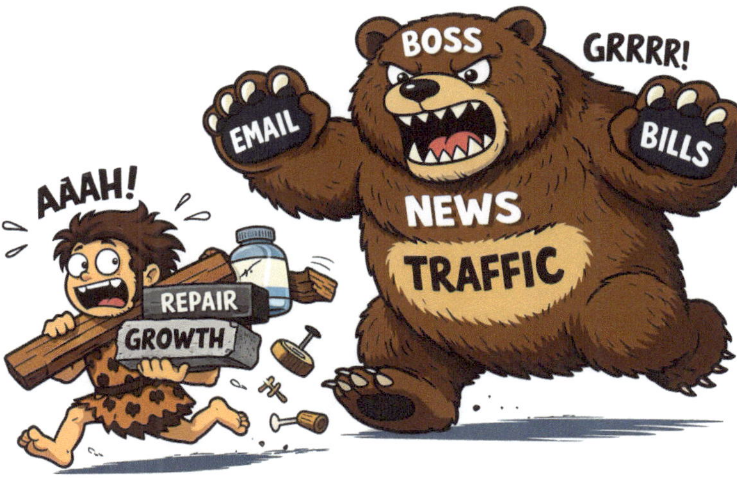

Your body was built for short bursts of stress not a permanent bear chase.

If you're having a sugary coffee drink in the morning and a dessert or soda in the afternoon, which is an extremely normal American routine, you're suppressing your testosterone twice a day, every day.

Over time, this isn't a temporary dip. It becomes your baseline. You wonder why you're tired, unmotivated, foggy, and gaining weight. Nobody tells you that the Frappuccino is stealing your energy currency.

The Testosterone Thief

What Sugar Does to Your Mood It doesn't stop at testosterone.

Researchers looked at 40 studies covering 1.2 million people and found that high sugar intake was associated with a 21% increased risk of depression.

That's not a small effect. That's a 21% higher chance of depression, from diet alone.

Here's how it works: sugar spikes your blood glucose. Then it crashes. The crash triggers your stress hormones. Stress hormones trigger cravings, for more sugar, more fast food, more of whatever gives quick relief. Inflammation rises. Your brain's chemistry shifts. Your mood follows.

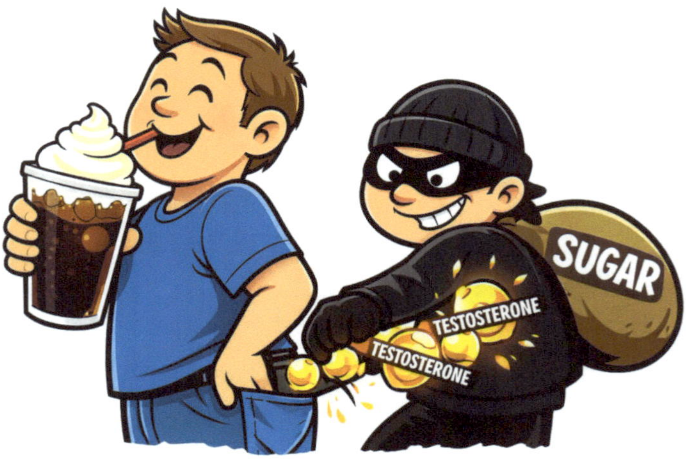

**One sugary drink drops testosterone 25 percent for two hours.
Do it every day and you're being robbed blind.**

This is the vicious cycle:

Stress → sugar craving → sugar → blood sugar crash → inflammation → worse mood → more stress → more sugar craving.

Round and round. The hamster wheel keeps spinning.

And if you're also sleep-deprived (see Chapter 5), also not exercising (see Chapter 6), also eating 60% ultra-processed food, the cycle spins faster.

The Hormonal Voltage Problem Your body runs on hormones the way a building runs on electricity. Testosterone, estrogen, thyroid hormone, cortisol, insulin, these are the voltage signals that keep every system running.

When the voltage is right, things work. Your brain is sharp. Your energy is stable. Your weight stays in range. Your mood is solid.

When the voltage drops or swings wildly, everything dims. Brain fog sets in. Energy crashes. Weight creeps up for reasons that don't make obvious sense. Mood becomes unpredictable.

This is what happens with chronic stress plus high sugar intake plus poor sleep. It's not just one hormone going wrong. It's the whole voltage system flickering.

The fix isn't one magic pill. It's fixing the inputs, and one of the cheapest, most powerful inputs is completely free.

The Free Fix: Morning Light Ten to thirty minutes of outdoor light before 10am resets your cortisol rhythm.

That's it. Stand outside in the morning. No sunglasses. No glass window in between. Just daylight on your eyes and skin.

Your eyes have special receptors that detect the specific wavelength of morning light and send a signal to your brain's master clock, the suprachiasmatic nucleus (su-pra-ky-az-MAT-ik, or just call it the "body clock"). This signal tells your cortisol to peak in the morning (when you want it) and drop in the evening (when you want to sleep).

Without morning light, your cortisol rhythm gets blurry. You wake up groggy. You crash in the afternoon. You can't fall asleep at night. And the whole stress system runs hotter than it should.

Ten minutes. Outside. Before 10am. It's free, and it works better than most sleep medications.

The Vicious Cycle

This Is Not in Your Head One more thing before we move on.

If you feel anxious, depressed, foggy, and exhausted, and your doctor has run labs and said you're "fine", it is very easy to start believing the problem is you. Your attitude. Your willpower. Your mental strength.

It's not.

It's biochemistry.

Chronically high cortisol physically damages mitochondria. Low testosterone physically affects your brain's dopamine system. Chronic inflammation physically disrupts the neurons that

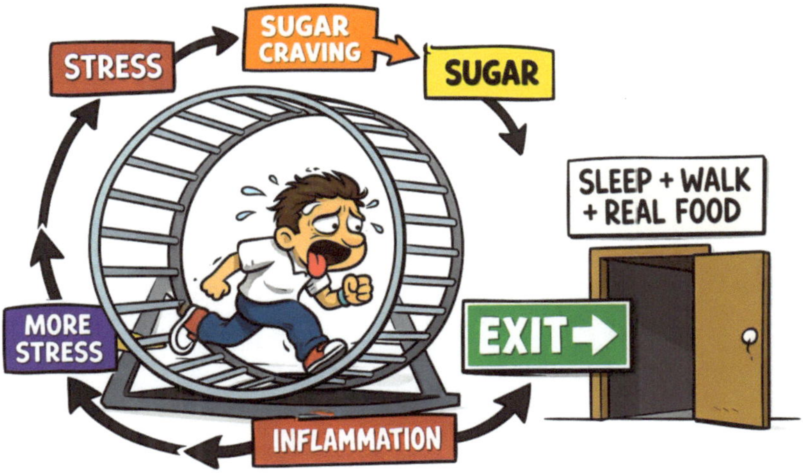

regulate mood. These are not character flaws. They are cellular conditions with cellular causes.

You are not broken. You are underpowered. And power can be restored.

The Simple Version

- Chronic stress keeps cortisol elevated. High cortisol puts your mitochondria in "survive" mode instead of "repair" mode. The power plants stop maintaining themselves.
- One sugary drink drops testosterone by 25% for two hours. Sugar also raises depression risk by 21% (from a study of 1.2 million people). These are connected.
- The stress-sugar-inflammation-bad mood cycle is a loop. You have to change the inputs to exit the loop.
- Morning light (10-30 minutes outside before 10am) resets your

cortisol rhythm. It's free and it works. Start there.

Chapter 9

The UCOS System: Fixing Things in the Right Order

Most people who feel lousy want to go straight to the advanced stuff. The exotic peptides. The IV drips. The special supplements nobody's heard of.

That's like bolting a racing spoiler onto a car with four flat tires, no oil, and a cracked engine block, and then wondering why it doesn't go faster.

You have to fix things in the right order. That's what the UCOS system is about.

What Is UCOS? UCOS stands for Ultimate Cellular Optimization System. It's the framework that ties together everything in this book.

It's not magic. It's not complicated. It's a checklist. A very specific, very ordered checklist, because the order matters.

Picture a staircase. Four steps. You cannot skip a step. You cannot jump from the ground to Step 4. You have to climb.

Most people are trying to step from the ground directly to the fourth step, wondering why they keep falling.

The UCOS Staircase

Step 1: Fix the Terrain Before anything else, you fix the terrain. This means your daily habits. Your inputs. The environment your cells live in.

Sleep. Food. Movement. Stress. Toxin exposure.

Here's the honest truth: for about half the people who do Step 1 and nothing else, just fix their sleep, eat more real food, walk daily, and manage their stress, they feel dramatically better. No supplements. No advanced tools. Just the terrain.

Because the terrain is where your cells live. If the terrain is broken, nothing else works well. You can take the most expensive supplements in the world, but if you're sleeping five hours a night and eating fast food twice a day, you are putting premium fuel into a car that has no oil in the engine.

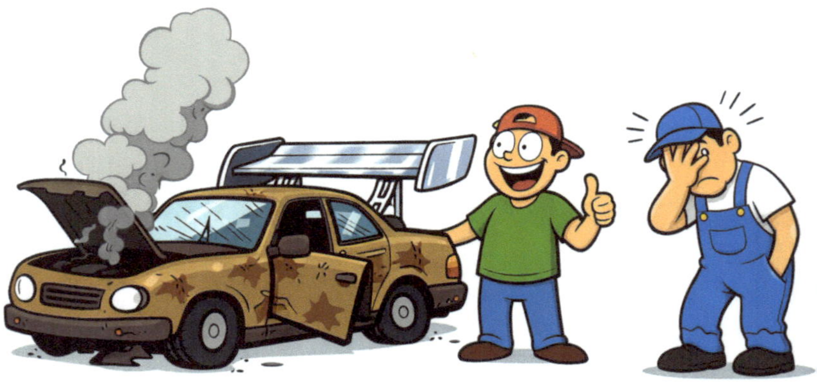

This is what it looks like when you take peptides but don't sleep, eat garbage, and never exercise.

So: Step 1.

Sleep 7 to 9 hours. Stop eating 3 hours before bed. Get 10 to 30 minutes of morning light. Walk 30 minutes a day. Eat a palm of protein at every meal. Drink water. Stop eating processed sugar like it's a hobby.

Do that for four weeks. Then and only then, move to Step 2.

Step 2: Fill the Gaps Even people who eat well and sleep well often have gaps. Specific nutrients that their power plants need and aren't getting enough of.

This is where targeted support comes in. And this is where the three products from Best365 Labs fit into the system. Not as magic, not as shortcuts, as tools to fill the specific gaps in your cellular toolkit.

Mito365, The Morning Power Plant Fuel

Your power plants need specific ingredients to run well. NAD+ (nicotinamide adenine dinucleotide, just say "NAD") is one of the most important. It's a molecule your cells use to convert food into energy. After age 40, NAD+ levels drop by about 50%. By age 60, they're down by two-thirds.

CoQ10 (coenzyme Q10) is another one. Think of it as the spark plug inside your power plant. Without it, the plant can't ignite properly.

PQQ (pyrroloquinoline quinone, just say "PQQ") helps grow new mitochondria. And methylene blue, yes, the stuff that turns your pee blue, is a powerful antioxidant that protects your power plants from oxidative damage.

Mito365 puts all of these in one morning formula. It's the power plant upgrade. You take it in the morning because that's when your body needs energy production to ramp up.

Think of it this way: you've been running your car on fumes. Mito365 is the oil change, the new spark plugs, and a tank of premium fuel, all at once.

Restore365, The Overnight Repair Crew

You learned in Chapter 5 that sleep is when your cells do their heaviest repair work. But repair requires the right tools.

GABA (gamma-aminobutyric acid, just say "GABA") is your brain's main calming signal. When GABA is working, your brain quiets down at night. When it's low, your mind races even when you're exhausted.

Melatonin at the right dose, 600 micrograms, not the massive 10-milligram horse pill at the pharmacy, is a powerful antioxidant that protects your mitochondria while you sleep. It's not a sedative. It's a signal that says, "Night shift starts now."

Magnesium glycinate helps relax muscles, calm the nervous system, and activate the ATP your cells are trying to use. (Remember: ATP without magnesium doesn't work. Mg-ATP is what your body actually runs on.)

Restore365 is the overnight repair crew. You take it in the evening. It closes the city down so the repair workers can come out.

Activate365, The Cellular Cleanup Crew

You know about autophagy, the garbage truck that clears out broken cell parts. And mitophagy, the garbage truck specifically for broken power plants.

Activate365 contains spermidine, a compound found in wheat germ and aged cheeses that powerfully triggers autophagy. It tells your body to start the cleanup process.

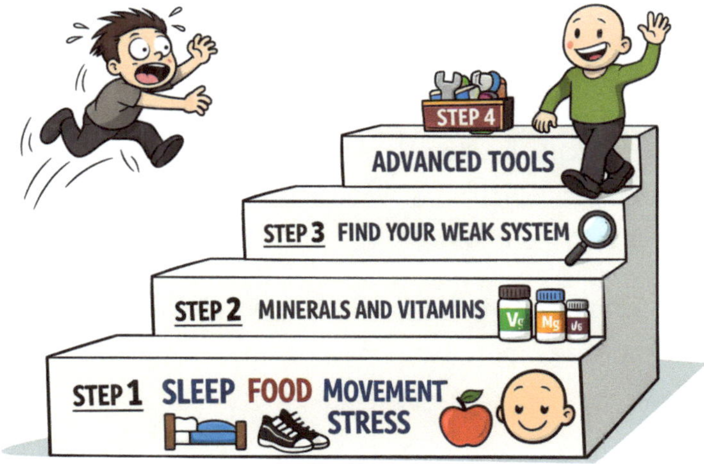
STEP 4
ADVANCED TOOLS
STEP 3 FIND YOUR WEAK SYSTEM
STEP 2 MINERALS AND VITAMINS
STEP 1 SLEEP FOOD MOVEMENT STRESS

It also contains quercetin and fisetin, two compounds that target zombie cells. Remember zombie cells from Chapter 3? The old, damaged cells that refused to die and instead just leaked inflammatory chemicals onto their neighbors? Quercetin and fisetin tell those zombie cells that the party is over.

Activate365 is the garbage truck plus the demolition crew. You take it in the morning or midday, especially during your fasting window, because that's when your body is most primed for cleanup.

The Three Bottles

Step 3: Find Your Weakest System Once the terrain is fixed and the nutrient gaps are filled, most people feel significantly better. But some people have a system that's specifically weak, and finding it lets you target your effort.

The UCOS model identifies five systems:

The Energy System, Are your power plants producing enough ATP? Signs of weakness: fatigue that doesn't improve with sleep, afternoon crashes, low motivation, struggling to recover from exercise.

The Structural System, Does your body hold together? Signs of weakness: joint pain, slow healing from cuts or injuries, easy bruising, back pain, poor posture.

The Brain and Mood System, Are your signals getting through clearly? Signs of weakness: brain fog, poor memory, mood instability, difficulty concentrating, depression or anxiety.

The Immune System, Is your security system working? Signs of weakness: getting sick often, slow recovery from illness, allergies that are getting worse, slow healing.

The Hormone System, Are your hormones stable? Signs of weakness: low libido, unexplained weight gain, hot flashes, mood swings, low testosterone, thyroid issues.

Identifying your weakest system tells you what to focus on in Step 4.

Step 4: Advanced Tools, But Only After 1-3 Are Solid

Peptide therapy. Hormone optimization. IV nutrient infusions. Personalized genetic testing. Advanced imaging.

These tools are real. They work. And they are dramatically more effective when your foundation is solid.

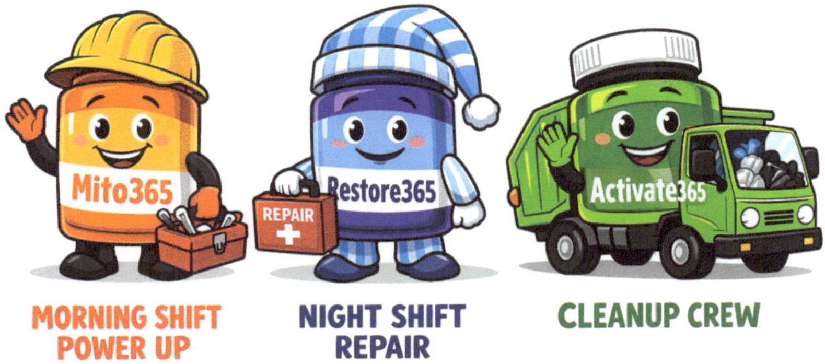

Power up. Repair. Clean up. Every day. That's the system.

The problem is that most people want to start here. They want the fancy tool. The injection. The drip.

A peptide injection in a body that sleeps 5 hours a night, eats sugar twice a day, and never exercises is like putting a spoiler on a broken car. It might look impressive. It will not go faster.

The Spoiler on a Broken Car

Fix the terrain. Fill the gaps. Find your weak system. Then, and only then, add the advanced tools. In that order.

The Loop, Not the Line Here's the most important thing about UCOS: it's not a one-time fix. It's a loop.

Test → Fix → Retest → Refine.

You get labs. You identify what's low or off. You take steps to fix it. You test again in 90 days to see if it worked. You adjust.

This is what real optimization looks like. Not one dramatic intervention. An ongoing, evidence-based loop that keeps your cells dialed in as your life changes, as you age, as seasons shift.

Your body is not a broken appliance you fix once and forget. It's a system that needs monitoring, maintenance, and occasional adjustment. The good news is that the monitoring is a simple blood draw, the maintenance is mostly lifestyle, and the adjustment gets easier the longer you do it.

The Simple Version

- UCOS is a four-step system: Fix the terrain (sleep, food, movement, stress) → Fill the gaps (Mito365, Restore365, Activate365) → Find your weak system → Add advanced tools.
- Do them in order. The spoiler does nothing if the engine is broken.
- Mito365 powers your morning. Restore365 repairs your overnight. Activate365 cleans up the debris. All three work together as a daily system.
- UCOS is a loop: Test → Fix → Retest → Refine. It never ends. That's the point.

Chapter 10

The 90-Day Reboot: Your Action Plan

Ninety days. Three phases. Each one builds on the last.

You will feel different. Not "a little better." Different. The kind of different where you tell a friend what you've been doing and they start asking for the list.

A Quick Look Back Before You Look Ahead You started this book learning that you have 37 trillion cells, each with power plants inside. Those power plants make the energy that runs every single function in your body, your brain, your muscles, your immune system, your mood, your metabolism.

When the power plants slow down, everything slows down. You get tired. You get foggy. You gain weight. Your hormones drop. Your sleep gets worse. Your mood tanks. And your doctor runs a blood panel that says you're "normal", because standard

medicine only checks if you've crashed, not if you're underpowered.

This whole book has been about one thing: giving your power plants back what they've been missing. In the right order. At the right time.

Here is that order, laid out in 90 days.

The 90-Day Road Map

Month 1 (Weeks 1-4): Fix the Foundation You cannot build on a bad foundation. This month is not about supplements. It's not about advanced tools. It's about giving your cells the conditions they need to start doing their jobs.

Most people feel meaningfully better just from Month 1. Sleep, sunlight, movement, protein, these are not boring basics. They are the most powerful cellular interventions that exist.

Sleep: 7 to 9 Hours

Pick a bedtime and stick to it. Your body's repair crew works on a schedule. If you keep changing when they're supposed to show up, they never get organized.

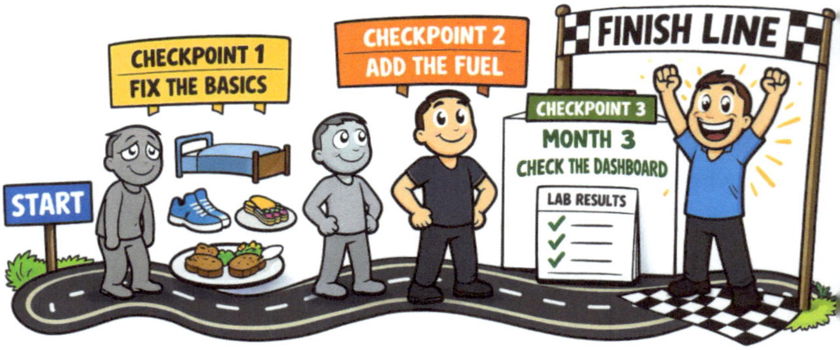
START
CHECKPOINT 1
FIX THE BASICS
CHECKPOINT 2
ADD THE FUEL
CHECKPOINT 3
MONTH 3
CHECK THE DASHBOARD
LAB RESULTS
FINISH LINE

Keep your room dark and cool. Darkness triggers melatonin. Cool temperature supports deep sleep. Both are non-negotiable for your repair window.

Stop eating 3 hours before bed. When food is in your gut, your body is in digestion mode. Digestion and deep repair don't run at the same time. Give yourself the window.

Morning Light: 10 to 30 Minutes

Get outside within an hour of waking up. No sunglasses. Just daylight. This resets your cortisol rhythm, sharpens your body clock, and sets up your sleep quality for that night.

It's free. It takes 10 minutes. Do it every day.

Movement: 30 Minutes of Zone 2 Walking

Walk fast enough that you can talk but you'd rather not. Every day. 30 minutes.

You don't have to do it all at once. Two 15-minute walks count. Three 10-minute walks count. The goal is to flip the mitochondrial biogenesis switch and get the garbage truck rolling.

Protein: A Palm at Every Meal

Breakfast, lunch, dinner, every meal gets a palm-sized portion of protein. Eggs, chicken, beef, fish, Greek yogurt, cottage

cheese, shrimp. It doesn't matter which, as long as it had a face or came from something that did.

This is not optional. Your cells rebuild themselves from protein. Without it, there are no building materials. The construction site shuts down.

Stop Eating 3 Hours Before Bed (and start your overnight fast)

This one does double duty. It improves your sleep quality. And it starts your body's cleanup window. Even a 12-hour overnight fast, say, done eating by 8pm and not eating again until 8am, activates your cleanup systems. The garbage truck finally gets a route.

Water

Drink half your body weight in ounces per day. A 180-pound person needs 90 ounces, about 11 cups. Your mitochondria need water to function. Your kidneys need water to clear waste. Your joints need water to move. Start here.

Month 2 (Weeks 5-8): Add the Support You've spent a month fixing the terrain. Your sleep is better. You're moving every day. You're eating more protein. Your body is ready to use the tools you're about to add.

Start Mito365, Morning

Take Mito365 in the morning, with or shortly after breakfast. Your power plants are ramping up for the day. Give them the NAD+, CoQ10, PQQ, and methylene blue they've been missing.

Think of this as finally changing the oil and installing new spark plugs in an engine that's been running rough for years. You may feel the difference within a few weeks. Some people feel it sooner.

Start Restore365, Evening

Take Restore365 in the evening, 30 to 60 minutes before bed. GABA calms the nervous system. Melatonin at 600 micrograms signals the repair window, without the grogginess that comes from the mega-doses at the pharmacy. Magnesium glycinate relaxes your muscles and activates your ATP.

Your sleep quality should improve. And better sleep means a more effective repair window, which means more energy the next day. It compounds.

Start Activate365, Morning or Midday

Take Activate365 in the morning or at midday, ideally during your fasting window if possible. Spermidine triggers autophagy. Quercetin and fisetin clear zombie cells. Your cleanup crew finally gets to do its job.

Before and After, Cells Edition

Add Resistance Training: 2 Sessions Per Week

By now, daily walking is a habit. Add two resistance training sessions per week. These can be at a gym, at home with dumbbells, or with bodyweight, push-ups, squats, lunges, rows.

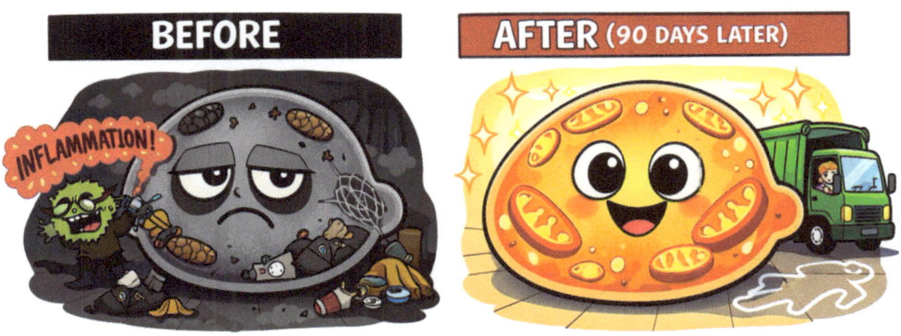

Same body. Same genes. Different inputs. 90 days.

Work your whole body over the two sessions. Keep it simple. The goal is to flip the mTOR switch, tell your muscles to grow, and maintain your hormonal voltage.

Expand Your Eating Window to 8 to 10 Hours

If you stopped eating 3 hours before bed in Month 1, you're already doing a partial fast. Now tighten it a little more. Aim to eat all your meals within an 8 to 10 hour window. This means 14 to 16 hours of overnight fasting.

That 14 to 16 hour window is when your AMPK switch is fully on, cleanup mode, fat-burning mode, repair mode. This is not a diet.

It's just letting your body alternate between building and cleaning, the way it was always designed to.

Month 3 (Weeks 9-12): Test and Refine By now, you feel different. Let's prove it with data, and use the data to keep getting better.

Get Labs Done

Ask your doctor for these specific tests:

• RBC magnesium, not serum magnesium. Serum magnesium looks normal even when your cells are depleted. You want the RBC test. • Homocysteine, the marker that shows whether your methylation system (your body's software update process) is working. • Vitamin D (25-OH), most people are low, and vitamin D is critical for immune function, mood, and hormone production. • Zinc, supports immune function, testosterone production, and wound healing. • Full hormone panel, testosterone (total and free), estrogen, thyroid (TSH, Free T3, Free T4), cortisol. These tests tell you which of your five systems is the weakest link. Energy. Structure. Brain and mood. Immune. Hormones. Once you know, you know where to focus.

Compare How You Feel to Day 1

Before you look at the labs, write down how you felt on Day 1. Your energy. Your brain clarity. Your sleep quality. Your mood. Your body composition. Your joint pain. Anything you were experiencing.

Then write down how you feel now. Most people are shocked by the gap.

The things they blamed on aging? Many of them are gone or dramatically improved. Not because they turned back time. Because they fixed a power shortage that had been building for years.

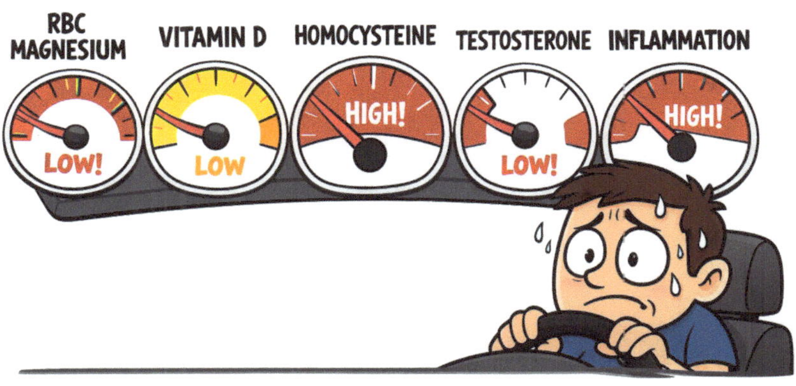

You check the dashboard on your car every time you drive.
When was the last time you checked the dashboard on your body?

The Lab Dashboard

Identify Your Weakest System

Based on your labs and how you feel, one or two of the five systems will stand out as needing more attention.

Low testosterone? That's the Hormone System. High homocysteine? That's the Brain System (methylation failure). Frequent illness? Immune System. Persistent fatigue despite good sleep and movement? Energy System. Joint pain that isn't improving? Structural System.

This is where you can add more targeted tools, specific nutrients, hormone support, or advanced interventions, with your doctor's guidance. But because you built the foundation first, those tools will work far better now than they ever would have at the start.

Adjust and Continue

The loop doesn't end after 90 days. It continues. You get labs every 3 to 6 months. You adjust based on what you find. You refine what's working. You address new weak points as they emerge.

This is not a burden. This is maintenance. The same maintenance you already give your car, your home, your phone. Your body deserves at least as much attention as your vehicle.

The Promise Here is the promise that started this book, and here is where it lands:

You are not "just getting older."

The fatigue is not inevitable. The brain fog is not permanent. The weight is not locked in. The mood crashes are not your personality. The low energy is not your ceiling.

These things happened because your 37 trillion power plants were running low, on the minerals they need, the sleep they require, the movement that builds them, the food that fuels them, and the cleanup that keeps them running clean.

You were not broken. You were underpowered.

And power can be restored.

In Chapter 1, we described your body as a city. A big, busy city where half the generators were sputtering, the lights were flickering, and nobody was checking the power plants.

After 90 days of doing this right, the lights start coming back on.

Not all at once. Not dramatically. But steadily. Reliably. Day by day, the city gets brighter.

Your brain runs at higher resolution. Your energy holds through the afternoon. The fat starts moving. Sleep becomes something you actually look forward to. Your mood stabilizes. You remember words again. You wake up before your alarm and don't mind.

This is not magic. This is mitochondria. And they've been waiting, all 37 trillion of them, for you to give them what they need.

Go fix the power plants.

The Simple Version

- Month 1: Fix the foundation. Sleep 7-9 hours. Morning light daily.

Walk 30 minutes a day. Protein at every meal. Stop eating 3

hours before bed. Drink water.

- Month 2: Add the tools. Mito365 in the morning. Restore365 in the evening. Activate365 morning or midday. Add resistance training twice a week. Tighten your eating window to 8-10 hours.
- Month 3: Test and refine. Get RBC magnesium, homocysteine, vitamin D, zinc, and a full hormone panel. Compare how you feel to Day 1. Find your weakest system. Adjust.
- The promise: What you blamed on aging was mostly a power shortage. Fix the inputs, restore the power, and discover what your body was actually capable of all along.

Want More Science?

For the full science, clinical protocols, and research behind everything in this book, read The Living Chip by Steven Warren, MD, DPA and Darren Lopez, MBA. Available on Amazon.

About the Products

The supplements mentioned in this book, Mito365, Restore365, and Activate365, are available at best365labs.com.

About the Authors

Steven Warren, MD, DPA is a triple-board-certified physician practicing in the Salt Lake City area.

Darren Lopez, MBA is the CEO of Best 365 Labs.

Get Help Here

If you read this book and still feel stuck, you do not have to figure it out alone. The 90-Day Reboot works for most people. For those who need more, that is what the clinic is for.

Regenerative Wellness Center

Salt Lake City area, Utah

Phone: 801-797-5901

Web: regwellness.com

Email: info@regwellness.com

Steven E. Warren, MD, DPA

Triple Board-Certified

Forty-five years in clinical practice

About the Author

Steven E. Warren, MD, DPA

Triple Board-Certified

Forty-five years of clinical practice in the Salt Lake City area. Triple Board-Certified in Family Medicine and Preventive Medicine, Addiction Medicine, and Hospice and Palliative Medicine. Certified Functional Medicine Practitioner and Independent Medical Examiner. Founder of the Regenerative Wellness Center, where the focus is restoring cellular function through evidence-based, regenerative protocols.

Author of The Living Chip (the clinical companion to this book), plus multiple books and clinical protocols in regenerative wellness, longevity, and spine care.

Regenerative Wellness Center

Salt Lake City area, Utah

Phone: 801-797-5901

Web: regwellness.com

Email: info@regwellness.com

About the Co-Author

Darren Lopez, MBA

Darren Lopez brings a business and operations lens to medical publishing and patient education. His work focuses on translating clinical complexity into materials patients can actually use. He co-authored this book to make sure the science stays clear without becoming watered down.

www.ingramcontent.com/pod-product-compliance
Lightning Source LLC
Chambersburg PA
CBHW041307210926
51847CB00005B/53
9781972800003